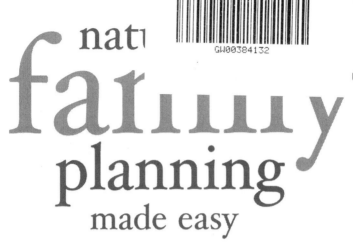

natural

family

planning

made easy

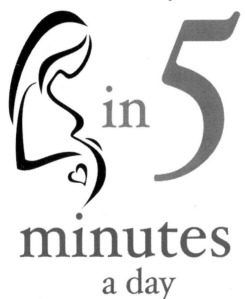

in 5

minutes

a day

KATE EVANS SCOTT

KL PRESS

DISCLAIMER

This book is dedicated to everyone who seeks to live their healthiest life.

ACKNOWLEDGMENTS

Thank You to our friends and family for your encouragement. Your support has been the cornerstone of this creative process.

A special thanks also goes out to you the reader ~ we are grateful to be sharing this journey to health and happiness together with you.

CONTENTS

CHAPTER 1

CHAPTER 2

CONTENTS

CHAPTER 3

CHAPTER 4

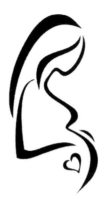

NATURAL FAMILY PLANNING MADE EASY IN JUST FIVE MINUTES A DAY

Natural Family Planning (NFP) is much more than just a form of birth control. It goes way beyond simply preventing pregnancy. NFP is an incredible opportunity for women to get in tune with their bodies... to understand their fertility cycle, the very core of their feminine self.

The practice of NFP also encourages couples to know and understand each other more intimately, not just on a sexual level, or on a superficial level. A woman and her husband embark on this journey together, planning carefully, abstaining together, and enjoying their rewards knowing fully that they are in control of their lives.

Beyond pregnancy prevention, NFP is used by many couples to help start a family. More often than not, the same couple will use NFP for different reasons as their marriage grows. You will likely start out using NFP to prevent pregnancy, and later use the information you've gathered to start your family or space your pregnancies. That's one of the many beauties of the method.

While you and your partner may just be learning about it, Natural Family Planning (NFP) isn't a new concept by any means. Nor was it effectively "invented" by the Catholic Church, as is the popular assumption. Women had been using the rhythm of their fertility cycle to control conception for ages before certain clergy began to endorse it. However, it *was* from within the constructs of Catholicism that our most modern and widely-used forms of NFP were conceived and developed.

Before we look at the basic how-to of Natural Family Planning, it's important to understand the concept's deep roots in the time line of humanity.

> "If you don't know where you are going, you'll end up someplace else."
>
> — Yogi Berra

HISTORY OF
NATURAL FAMILY PLANNING

In modern times, a woman's menstrual cycle has become a taboo topic. For far too many women, discussion of their period is shameful and embarrassing. They don't want to talk about fertility and their bodies have become "sexualized" to the point that any discussion of it is considered dirty and shameful. We tend to look at menstruation as a horrible, painful, frustrating time of the month that we'd rather avoid if at all possible. Modern women often don't understand their changing physical and emotional states as their bodies turn from fertile to infertile and back again... nor do they want to.

Instead of being celebrated as the bearers of life, today's women are often labeled as "PMS-ing" (or, acting irrational and emotional), as popular media and sociocultural norm depict women's cycles as something to either ignore or abhor. Television commercials and print ads tell women to keep performing all of their regular activities as if nothing were different... as if they didn't feel bloated, headachey, cramped, or fatigued... as if the miracle of their fertility cycle weren't changing them both physically and emotionally. A woman's period is an inconvenience to be dealt with secretly (or discreetly).

Drugs are developed and manufactured to help manage mood swings, clear up the cyclical acne, and ease sore muscles. You can buy products to take care of vaginal dryness or increase your low libido... you can buy all kinds of lotions, pills, and ointments to manage the "symtoms" of your cycle, but no-one is telling women how to listen to and respect the miracle that's happening within their bodies.

At least, it seems like no-one is... but that isn't completely true!

Couples who practice NFP learn to talk openly about a woman's fertility cycle. They begin to gain a new respect for the female body. Men begin to understand their wife's emotional state-- why one day a sideways comment might earn a laugh, and then another day, the same comment could start a fight. Husband and wife empower one another. They rely on each other. These couples learn to look for intimacy on a deeper level much different than the kind found in the bedroom.

With the help of trained practitioners, couples can not only build their families according to their own design, they can build a stronger foundation for that family in the form of a healthier, more loving relationship.

BRIEF HISTORY OF WOMEN AND FERTILITY

There is nothing more powerful than truly understanding your own body.

For thousands of years, our greatest grandmothers knew their bodies on an intimate level that we likely could not even comprehend in the midst of the hustle and bustle of our fast-paced techno-world. We are fighting a constant barrage of artificial input, a social message that says femininity means weakness, and cultural stigma equating menses with uncleanliness. Talking about your period is suddenly awkward... but it wasn't always so.

Prior to industrialization, when electric lights made it possible for us to rise before dawn and stay up all night, women's fertility cycles were more in sync with the natural world. Their menstrual cycles were more regular, and in fact were closely in line with the waning and waxing of the moon. I know it sounds a bit "mystical," but it's actually true. Often times, whole villages of women ovulated and menstruated at the same time.

There are, in fact, records of women during Biblical time (such as Jacob's wives, 1836 – 1689BC), gathering in tents during their menstruation—separated from the often physically exhausting routine and chores of daily life. This was a time of rest, a time to listen to and revere the incredible changes occurring in their bodies, a time to bond with other women and recover from the loss of blood. It was a time to quietly celebrate their womanhood.

During this time each month, mothers and daughters talked openly about menstruation, sex, and childbirth. For much of recorded civilization, women knew the signs and signals of their fertility cycle... that is, until discussing such things became taboo, and a woman's menstruation became "dirty." How did this happen? Well, it was a gradual shift that was reinforced by the earliest practice of many of the world's organized religions- such as Judaism, Islam, Hinduism, and Christianity. While this "ritual uncleanliness" (as it was referred to) is not necessarily an accepted association to today, the cultural stigma has remained.

Alongside religious conviction, the rise of patriarchal societies also worked toward repressing women's sexuality, which helped to stifle discussion (even amongst women) of their fertility and their bodies.

As civilization experienced a shift from a mainly matriarchal to a patriarchal society, the only way to ensure that land and money were passed down through the line of sons was to make absolutely sure that a woman remained monogamous. This caused a cultural clench on women's sexuality, which was accomplished largely through public shame... and even through public torture. Women could not, and should not, be in control of their own bodies. Knowledge was power, and in a patriarchal society, women with power were dangerous.

So, bit by bit, women lost their community of sisters in which to confide and share, and thus lost touch with their ability to understand their bodies on such an intimate level. Now, generations and generations later, this negative association with a woman's natural cycle is still leaving women confused, afraid, and ashamed of their own bodies.

A surprising result of practicing Natural Family Planning is that you and your partner will gain a new reverence for, and understanding of, your body and the potential for life that resides within you. This knowledge and understanding is very powerful, and can bond you and your husband in ways you'd never have imagined.

HISTORY OF NFP
IN THE CATHOLIC CHURCH

The Roman Catholic Church teaches that contraception goes against the will of God. It has long been their practice that intercourse is never to be separate from the openness to new life. In other words, sex is for procreation. Period.

However, Natural Family Planning is now endorsed by the church as a morally correct way of spacing out the birth of children during marriage. Why? Because the only acceptable form of birth control is abstinence. NFP is, indeed, a birth control method that incorporates periods of abstinence directly correlating with a woman's periods of naturally-occurring high or peak fertility.

The history of the Catholic view on contraception dates way back to the Teaching of the Twelve Apostles in 94 AD condemning contraception. Then, some 300 years later, St. Augustine claimed that any sexual intercourse which avoids the conception of offspring was "unlawful and shameful." So, the intent of copulation should always be procreation.

Then again in 1215 AD, St. Thomas Aquinas condemned any deliberate action to exclude potential offspring from the act of intercourse. This ideology was confirmed again and again by theologians of all faiths and popes throughout history until the beginning of the 20th century. It's not necessarily "preaching abstinence," but instead is essentially saying, "Have intercourse for the purpose of procreating."

It has always been clear that Catholicism only condoned sexual relationships as part of the human design to procreate. However, in the mid 1800's, a ruling from the church's Sacred Penitentiary addressed the topic of periodic abstinence to avoid pregnancy. In a statement delivered to confessors, the ruling stated that couples who had, on their own, begun the practice of periodic abstinence—especially if they had "legitimate reasons"—were not sinning by doing so.

This meant that intercourse could be avoided during fertile periods, and engaged in during infertile periods, thus paving the way for several different contemporary methods of Natural Family Planning utilized by both Catholics and non-Catholics today.

In 1951, Pope Pius XII officially approved periodic abstinence and the Calendar Method of NFP, and openly asked physicians to move forward in their research in this regard. However, a succession of popes continued to preach about openness to life when regarding sexual relations, clearly condemning artificial birth control.

Meanwhile, Catholic organizations and physicians continued to work tirelessly on perfecting various methods of encouraging or avoiding pregnancy based on the calendar, body temperature, and varied physical symptoms during a woman's fertility cycle. This was the inception of modern Natural Family Planning.

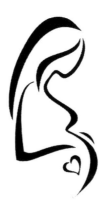

NATURAL FAMILY PLANNING TODAY!

Now, there are several different methods commonly used by couples either looking to avoid pregnancy or to conceive. Some methods are considered more effective than others, while some methods are simpler to follow. Some require special devices and other just a pen and paper. The key to using any method of NFP effectively is consistency... and you'll see why.

Before digging in, it's important to remember that every couple is different. You may find that you just don't want to know the science, you'd rather just know if having intercourse on this day will likely result in pregnancy. That's fine.

You may want to be more independent, dig into the research, and learn everything you can about your body. Go for it! OR, you might rather leave all that research to the professionals. It's okay to do that... that's what they're trained to do.

You might find a teacher and a method you click with right away, or you and your partner might go through a few before you find out what works for you. The most important thing is to stick with it until you find your fit—remember, your reproductive years are long, and you want them to be as happy as possible.

I've outlined a few of the most popular NFP methods being used today. Please keep in mind that this is a brief overview, and more research may be required prior to making a decision about your preferred method.

CALENDAR METHOD
(STANDARD DAYS METHOD)

Using this method, a woman can predict fertile days by charting and recording how long her menstrual cycle lasts. This will give her insight into which days she is fertile each month, and which days she is not.

HERE'S HOW IT WORKS: To predict the first day you are likely to be fertile (increased probability of pregnancy) in your new cycle, you will need to have cycle information from the last 8 – 12 months. This is crucial to the efficacy of this method—which means, yes, you'll need to abstain during that time.

Your cycle begins with the first day of your period and ends the day before your period beginning the next cycle. Mark these days clearly on your calendar.

Take the shortest menstrual cycle and subtract 18 days. When you start your next period, take that number and count forward on the calendar and this should be the first day that you are likely to be fertile in the upcoming cycle.

To predict the end of your fertile stretch, take the number of days in your longest cycle and subtract 11. Count forward on the calendar that number from the day you start your period.

It's a little bit confusing, so let me give you an example. Let's say you've charted your cycle for the past 9 cycles (around 8 – 9 months), and these are the numbers you derived:

CYCLE	FIRST	SECOND	THIRD	FOURTH	FIFTH
DAYS/CYCLE	27	28	28	29	27

CYCLE	SIXTH	SEVENTH	EIGHTH	NINTH
DAYS/CYCLE	29	28	27	28

You are just starting your period for your tenth cycle, and it's January 3rd.

To determine when you will likely be most fertile in this cycle, follow this equation:

27 (the shortest cycle) – 18 = 9

To determine when your fertility period will likely end, follow this equation:

29 (your longest cycle) – 11 = 18

Start counting forward on the calendar for 9 days, including the day your menstruation begins, and mark the first day of your fertility period. Count 18 days from the first day of your menstruation to mark the end of your fertility period:

Sunday	Monday	Tuesday	Wednesday	Thursday	Friday	Saturday
			1	2	ONE **3** (MENSES START)	TWO **4**
5 THREE	**6** FOUR	**7** FIVE	**8** SIX	**9** SEVEN	**10** EIGHT	**(11)** NINE
(12) TEN	**(13)** ELEVEN	**(14)** TWELVE	**(15)** THIRTEEN	**(16)** FOURTEEN	**(17)** FIFTEEN	**(18)** SIXTEEN
(19) SEVENTEEN	**(20)** EIGHTEEN	21	22	23	24	25
26	27	28	29	30	31	

So, in this example, the likely period of high fertility for the upcoming cycle would be from January 11th- January 20th. If you are trying to avoid pregnancy, you would NOT engage in intercourse during those ten days of that cycle.

However, if you are trying to conceive, those days would be the time to try!

5 MINUTES A DAY: Record your menstrual cycle onto the calendar. *Okay, so this may not even take five minutes!*

The benefit of this method is in its simplicity. All you need to do is track when you're menstruating and write it down on the calendar—with a little bit of simple math, you've got your chart. *The drawback is that this method has the most room for error. It's advisable to use this method in conjunction with one of the other methods of NFP.*

BASAL BODY TEMPERATURE METHOD

This method of NFP takes a little bit more work, and relies on the science of the body. Your basal body temperature is exactly as it sounds—the baseline. It's your body's resting temperature, and can be most accurately measured right when you wake up in the morning.

By tracking and recording your basal body temperature for a few months, you can reasonably predict when you will be fertile in the upcoming cycle.

HERE'S HOW IT WORKS: Your basal body temperature is typically between 96°F and 98°F *before ovulation.* After ovulation, your basal body temperature rises about one degree. As you can imagine, this slight discrepancy is difficult to detect and really necessitates a basal body thermometer.

In order to follow this method, you will need to take your basal body temperature every morning as soon as you wake—at as close to the same time as possible. Your fertility is at its highest 2-3 days after your temperature peaks, and drops 3 days after it has risen.

If you are using this method, you will need to purchase or download a basal body temperature chart and purchase a basal body thermometer. After recording your temperature fluctuations for several months, you should be able to predict your periods of fertility.

5 MINUTES A DAY: Measure and record your basal body temperature first thing upon waking. It helps to keep your chart and thermometer right next to your bed so your measurements are as accurate as possible!

CERVICAL MUCUS METHOD (CMM) OR OVULATION METHOD (OM)

This method is a little more "hands-on," and requires you to be very comfortable with your body. CMM relies on observation of the cervical mucus, which changes as a woman goes through her cycle. There are a variety of approaches to observing and charting these changes, including those taught by:

- Billings Ovulation Method Association—USA
- Creighton Model FertiltyCare™ Centers
- Family of the Americas

Each of the methods requires daily observation and charting of the color and thickness of your cervical mucus, or of the sensation surrounding the vulva, depending on the specific method you choose.

HERE'S HOW IT WORKS: When your menstruation ends, most women experience 2 – 3 "dry days," or days when no mucus is present in the cervix area. There will be no discharge and intercourse during this time could be painful without additional lubricant. These few dry days are likely to be infertile—days when you are unlikely to conceive.

As your body prepares an egg for release (ovulation), more mucus is produced. This mucus is generally white or yellow colored and sticky to the touch. When your body is producing this cervical mucus, it's more likely that you'll conceive, while it's not yet the most fertile time in your cycle.

Just before you ovulate, the most mucus is produced. This mucus is thick, clear, and slippery—similar in color and texture to raw egg whites. A woman's body produces this mucus to prepare for intercourse, and thus, conception. This is the absolute most fertile time in your cycle, and the time that you are most likely to get pregnant.

After three or four days of slippery, thick mucus, you are likely to produce much less mucus. What is produced is dark and cloudy in color and a bit sticky, rather than slippery. This is followed by a couple of dry days before the onset of your next menstruation. During this time between slippery and your next period, it's unlikely that you will become pregnant.

This method, when discerned correctly, is very accurate and based on real-time physiology as well as charted cycles for better indication.

5 MINUTES A DAY: With your fingers or a tissue, check your cervical discharge several times throughout each day and record it on a calendar or chart. Mark your days with code words such as "Dry, Sticky/Cloudy, or Slippery/Thick/Clear."

SYMPTO-THERMAL METHOD (STM)

This method involves cross-checking multiple fertility indicators in order to achieve a more accurate prediction of fertility. STM combines the practice of checking and recording cervical mucus and charting basal body temperature.

Other optional indicators may also be checked, depending on which organization you're learning from and working with—as several huge organizations dedicated to the practice of STM are in operation today: Couple to Couple League and Northwest Family Services are two of the largest.

Some practitioners of STM will also check and record such secondary fertility signs as breast tenderness and/or slight pain around one ovary.

HERE'S HOW IT WORKS: Follow both the Basal Body Temperature and Cervical Mucus Methods.

5 MINUTES A DAY: Measure and record your basal body temperature, and check and record your cervical mucus several times throughout each day. You may also check secondary fertility signs such as breast tenderness and/or pain around one ovary.

> "Condoms aren't completely safe. A friend of mine was wearing one and got hit by a bus."
>
> — Bob Rubin

SYMPTO-HORMONAL METHOD (SHM)

This method not only uses observation of several fertility indicators, it adds a special device called an ovulation predictor kit (OPK) or fertility monitor. The monitor detects reproductive hormones levels present in a woman's urine.

HERE'S HOW IT WORKS: There are six days of fertility during a woman's menstrual cycle—ovulation day and the five days before. This is called the *fertile window*. During this time, two female reproductive hormones are produced called estrogen and LH. The OPK measures the urinary metabolites of those two reproductive hormones to help you determine your fertile window.

The results will come out Low, High, or Peak. If you're trying to avoid pregnancy, you want to avoid having sex during the high and peak days. Of course, if your goal is to conceive, intercourse is advisable during peak days!

While it looks simple, the biggest problem with this method is that it's a bit easy to goof it up—you can hold the OPK in the urine stream for too long, for example, resulting in a greater number of High results. Also, there's a bit of a complicated equation to figuring out the fertility cycle in order to properly read the test results. Hormone levels are going to be different for women just having given birth or who are breast feeding, who have irregular periods or who are above and below a certain age.

If you're looking at using this system, you must purchase the OPK and read all instructions thoroughly. You should also take a class on the Marquette Method or another Sympto-Hormonal system in order to fully understand how to measure and chart your hormone levels. It's important not to go it alone... that's why there are certified NFP practitioners to help guide you through this process.

5 MINUTES A DAY: Test your urine with the OPK and record results. Check and record your cervical mucus. *By testing both the hormone levels and analyzing the cervical mucus, this method doubles up for better accuracy.*

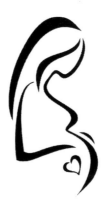

CHOOSING THE RIGHT METHOD FOR YOU

Now that you've had a quick overview of the various methods, it's time to pick the one that's right for you and your partner. I've given you an at-a-glance guide to help you match your personality, goals, and ____ with the NFP method that will best meet your needs!

Most people who practice NFP use either a combination of CMM and BBT (Sympto-Thermal), Hormones and CMM (Sympto-Hormonal), or CMM. The Standard Day Method alone is a bit risky and should only be used if you are truly are open to new life.

THE SYMPTO-THERMAL METHOD
is right for you if:

- You wake up (or could wake up) at about the same time every single morning (within ½ hour), and sleep for at least a continuous three hours prior to waking.

- You're a super-careful person who likes the idea of always having a backup.

- Avoiding pregnancy (or conceiving) are really important concerns... there's little flexibility there.

- You don't mind getting familiar with your vaginal secretions.

- You're thrifty—you don't want to spend more than about ten bucks on materials.

- You have a somewhat regular cycle, but are not necessarily interested in doing anything to regulate that.

Congratulations—you're perfect for the Sympto-Thermal Method! Here are some resources to get you started:

- **Couple-to-Couple League:**
  http://www.ccli.org/

- **Northwest Family Services:**
  http://www.nwfs.org/

- **Taking Charge of Your Fertility:**
  http://www.ovusoft.com/

DO NOT use this method if you get up really early during the week exhausted from broken sleep due to your cats waking you up all through the night, crash until noon on the weekends, hate the thought of touching your cervical mucus, and don't really mind if you get pregnant or not.

THE SYMPTO-HORMONAL METHOD
is right for you if:

- You don't mind peeing on a stick.

- You wake up within a couple of hours range each day (like, between 7:00am and 9:00am, for example).

- You and your partner would prefer not to have to rely mainly on charts to know if you can have sex—you'd rather have a monitor tell you.

- You don't mind spending a couple hundred dollars on "stuff" for your NFP.

- You are postpartum or breast feeding.

- You have an irregular cycle or special medical circumstances.

Awesome—the Sympto-Hormonal method might just be your model! Check out this resource to get you started. There's a ton of information here, including how to monitor your hormone levels when you have special circumstances:

- **Marquette Model:**
  http://nfp.marquette.edu/

DO NOT use this method if the thought of accidentally touching urine grosses you out, your sleep schedule is all over the place, and you don't have money to spend on date night let alone a couple hundred for equipment.

THE CERVICAL MUCUS METHOD
is right for you if:

- When do you get up in the morning? You'll know tomorrow, it's all over the place.

- You don't mind putting all your eggs in one basket, so to speak.

- You have a bit of money to spend if necessary, but you'd rather hold onto it in case of emergency.

- You don't mind observing your mucus a few times a day.

- Your periods are a bit irregular, and you'd love to "fix" them!

Sounds like CMM is right for you! There are a few different schools of CMM, so let me spell them out a bit more for you here so you can make the best choice possible.

BILLINGS METHOD OF CMM

The Billings Method was developed primarily as a method of avoiding pregnancy, but it has also been used effective to conceive. This method focuses on sensation at the vulva, and does not require you to touch the cervical mucus for its viscosity (thickness or stickiness). This could be good for you if you don't like touching body fluids.

When using this method, you'll make your observations as you go about your daily routine—no need to go into the rest room to take test samples! You'll learn about your own fertility cycle intimately, charting it in your own language and method that's easiest for you to understand and use.

The rules of this method are simple, and you will learn to identify your peak (corresponds to ovulation) through observation of vulvic sensation. While you can start out with a class or practitioner, the ultimate goal is for you to become independent of them. This means that the classes are heavy on the "science" of fertility. You can also do a lot of this research online. If you're not into studying science, and you'd rather have the support of a practitioner throughout your NFP practice, you may not want to use this method.

However, if you're squeamish about talking "sex" with men, the Billings method could be a relief—it's taught woman to woman.

DO NOT use this method if you would rather someone be there to guide you on your journey, start to finish; like to have backup for your backup; and would rather not study science-- you had enough of that in school thanks very much.

CREIGHTON MODEL FERTILITYCARE™

The Creighton Model is quite different from the Billings model in a few different ways. First off, the Creighton Model was designed as a method of achieving pregnancy, but it can also be used as a prevention method.

Focusing on the cervical mucus itself, you will be required to observe your vaginal discharge each time you use the rest room—at least several times a day.

Quite opposite of the Billings method, this method is standardized so that the practitioner you'll be working with throughout the process can easily understand your cycle. Then, your practitioner will devise the proper method specifically for you. This means that the paperwork is done for you, all the way down to the charts!

While you won't have to do a lot of scientific research using this method, you will be much more reliant on your practitioner/teacher—who is also a medical practitioner and will be in charge of your full reproductive care. This dependence on your practitioner takes the weight off of your shoulders and provides you with an instant network.

DO NOT use this method of CMM if you can't stand touching body fluid (or looking at it), would rather be independent than have to rely on anyone else for help, or do better using your own signs and charts—because maybe you just have a unique way of looking at things.

Here are some resources for you to check out before you make your decision:

- **Creighton Model FertilityCare System:** http://www.fertilitycare.org/
- **Billings Method:** http://www.boma-usa.org/
- **Family of the Americas:** https://www.familyplanning.net/

Cervical mucus is one of the most reliable real-time indicators of ovulation, making CMM an effective addition to any method of NFP.

"Someone's sitting in the shade today because someone planted a tree a long time ago."

— Warren Buffett

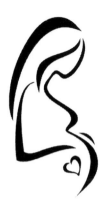

TIPS FOR QUICK AND EASY CHARTING

For any of the NFP methods, charting is the first step in the process—and it's incredibly important! So, you want to get it right... but you don't want it to be exhausting. In comes the internet (better living through technology). There are countless sources out there for downloading paper charts for each of the methods.

BASAL BODY TEMPERATURE CHARTS

http://www.contracept.org/nfpchart.php

http://www.babycenter.com/0_blank-bbt-chart_7069.bc

(This one also charts cervical mucus.)

SYMPTO-THERMAL METHOD (STM) CHARTS

http://www.nwfs.org/couples-a-singles/natural-family-planning/downloadable-chart.html

http://www.fertilityinstructor.com/paper.html

http://holistichormonalhealth.com/charts/

SYMPTO-HORMONAL METHOD (SHM) CHARTS

http://www.hormonalforecaster.com/download.aspx

You can also purchase charting apps for your Android or iPhone (iPad).

BILLINGS OVULATION METHOD CHARTING APP

https://itunes.apple.com/us/app/nfp-charting/id300767738?mt=8

SYMPTO-THERMAL METHOD ANDROID APP

- Fertility Friend

  http://www.fertilityfriend.com/android/

- myNFP

  https://itunes.apple.com/app/id466385600

BASAL BODY TEMPERATURE CHARTING APP

- Woman Calendar for Android
  https://itunes.apple.com/us/app/woman-calendar/
  id290591983?mt=8

If you don't see what you're looking for, keep looking. There are dozens of charting mobile apps, desktop programs, and downloadable charts to help you keep track of your fertility cycle. However, your first resource for charts should be your trained NFP practitioner (teacher), which you will find when you *take a class!* I can't stress enough the importance of starting out with a class in your chosen method.

Once you have your chart, follow these quick and simple tips for making the process of charting as easy as possible!

Keep your chart handy. If you're measuring basal body temperature, keep your chart and pen (or mobile device) and basal thermometer right next to your bed. If you're testing urine (hormonal) or checking cervical mucus, keep that chart close to the toilet in the rest room you most commonly use.

Stay organized. Keep a binder or folder containing all of your fertility information in a safe place that is easily accessible. Don't keep track of your fertility on your big family planning calendar. Not only could that be a bit awkward, your info could get lost amidst penned-in meetings and birthday reminders!

Use what works! Just because you started out with an app, doesn't mean you're married to it. If it's not working for you, try a new app or switch to a paper method. Just make sure you transfer or otherwise record your information so you can continue with your charting—nothing's worse than having to start all over!

Check with your teacher. Your NFP instructor is an invaluable resource… and some methods may require you to use their charting materials! In order to keep the process as smooth as possible, start out by asking your teacher which charting materials they suggest.

Talk to your partner. Remember, this is a "group effort." You'll be checking these charts together to determine when you can engage in and avoid sexual intercourse, so make sure you include him in the decisions. Is he more comfortable looking at apps, or reading paper charts? Making the choice together will help him feel more involved and encourage him to participate in the process.

Your charts are going to become a part of your daily routine, so just make sure you're prepared and making it as easy on yourself as possible—it's just five minutes a day, but you might as well make those five minutes a breeze.

GETTING THROUGH
THE ROUGH STUFF

Okay, as far as birth control methods go, NFP isn't the easiest possible route. It takes a lot more work than swallowing a pill every day. It's much more time-intensive than using prophylactics (condoms)... and it takes some amount of restraint and conviction on the part of both you and your partner.

So, why use it then? There are a number of reasons a couple might choose NFP over other types of birth control. The most common reason is one of religious conviction- primarily Catholic. However, statistically speaking, only about 5% of Catholic women utilize this method, as many Catholics have changed their belief regarding contraceptives... and others choose to always be open to receiving the gift of life.

Some couples choose to use NFP as a preventative method for health reasons—it's totally natural, so there are not the kinds of side-effects and hormone disruptions associated with it that you may experience with other female contraceptive methods. PLUS, when used correctly, it's just as effective as the pill. That's why you're going through this process, right? To understand how to use NFP correctly!

OR, you may be using NFP to PLAN a pregnancy! Getting pregnant is more difficult for some couples than others. Knowing when a woman is most fertile can help these couples plan intercourse at the time that conception is most likely.

I'm not going to lie to you—it's not always easy. Some people might go so far as to say that NFP, either for preventative or procreative purposes, "ruined their marriage!" It can make sex seem like a chore, always charting and planning and testing and observing. Then, there's the period of abstinence (for couples using it as a preventative) that lasts for a few days in the middle of each cycle. If you're not careful, the combination of these things can make you resentful, spiteful, withdrawn, and frustrated. Then there's that nagging thought that you just might still get pregnant, which can make sex a bit nerve-racking until you are really confident in your body and your method.

But I'll be the first one to say, if your marriage falters in the face of family planning, NFP didn't ruin your marriage—there was likely some deeper seeded issue brought to the forefront in the face of this new challenge. For some people, it's just easier to blame the method than to scrutinize themselves.

Ultimately, when you and your partner are both on board with NFP, you will develop a deeper and more nurturing relationship that can't be found in any other form of contraception, prescription pill, IUD, or in a condom. You two will become bonded as one as you forge your way through this basic life process—and you'll find joy, excitement, arousal, and satisfaction in one another both intimately and cognitively.

So, you've made the decision to use NFP, and it's time to get started! Here are a few tips to help you prepare yourself for the process, strengthen your conviction, and give you hope in times of weakness.

SIGN UP FOR CLASSES!

It is very important that you do not try to go it alone. Seek out a class specially designed to teach your chosen method and provide you with the support you need as you learn the ins-and-outs of NFP.

In fact, some methods require you to take a class because the teacher is integral in the process of individualizing your system. Remember, we're talking about your body, your family, and the potential of pregnancy... the more you know and the more support you have, the more power you have over your own life.

In addition to the organizations listed in the Resources section, here are a few that also offer NFP classes either on site or online. Some classes are local on site courses, others are internet-based, and still other organizations have chapters and locations all over the country or world. To find out more about each individual organization, check out the links provided.

NFP International (NFPI)

Website: http://www.nfpandmore.org

NFPI provides both clients and teachers a complete educational program in Sympto-Thermal Method (STM), also called the Cross-Check Method. Client education is online and support is offered via e-mail and phone. NFPI also offers master teacher programs via email as well as "Ecological Breast feeding" education.

Northwest Family Services (NWFS)

6200 SE King Road

Portland, OR 97222

Website: http://www.nwfs.org/

(503) 546-6377

(503) 546-9397 FAX

Email: service@nwfs.org

NWFS provides education in the Fertility Matters method (of STM), which uses cervical mucus detection and interpretation, basal body temperature charting, as well as changes in the cervix and secondary fertility signs.

They offer both client and teacher education in the SymptoPro method through correspondence via post, internet, and a combination of the two for those who request it. A charting app is made available, as well as a newsletter and a variety of other educational programs.

One More Soul NFP Directory

Web address: http://onemoresoul.com/nfp_by_cat/ NFP_Centers

One More Soul provides an interactive directory of NFP centers by city and state/Province in North America and Canada. Most of the centers listed offer on site classes, which can be beneficial if you are looking for a community and are comfortable talking about fertility in a group setting. The organization also offers many other programs and a wealth of information centered around the Catholic view of NFP.

SHOP AROUND

If you try one class or one method and you don't like it, try something else. There are a number to choose from, and each one will vary slightly based on several factors, including who is teaching it! It's really important for you to **like your teacher**, and work well with the method. This is not the fifth grade... and you're not stuck with who you get. If you are not clicking with your NFP instructor, or perhaps the vibe in the group feels a bit off, look for another class or switch to another instructor.

You should also be wary of instructors who are not willing to let you consider another method when either theirs isn't working well for you, or when you have medical complications that make charting for that method difficult. Some teachers get really gung-ho about their own approach and aren't willing to listen to alternatives. These people are extremists, and are narrow-minded, even to the detriment of your successful NFP experience. It's like they've sworn allegiance to one system, never to sway or falter. You won't survive with that kind of rigidity. You don't want that instructor. This is YOUR life, your body, your care... and you are the one who has to be completely comfortable with all aspects of your NFP, or it will drive you nuts... and you could ultimately fail either because the method wasn't best for you, or because you give up out of frustration. Don't let that happen.

START YOUR CHART!

Do it now. Are you just engaged? Thinking of getting engaged? Thinking of maybe finding a boyfriend? Start charting NOW! No matter what method you choose, the more records you have of your cycle and symptoms the more accurately and easily you'll be able to predict your fertile days. Sign up for the class, learn the method, and get going. Remember, you NEED at least 8 months of charting before intercourse... but in this case, more is better.

FORGET ABOUT IT

You know that whole thing about the 28 day cycle... well, that's not exactly accurate for every single woman. So when you get charting, don't worry if things jump around and the chart doesn't look exactly like you think it should. There is no "should." However, if you think something looks way out of line, that's the time you call on your friendly, carefully chosen NFP teacher to take a look. If there seems to be a medical issue that needs attention, they'll help you locate an NFP-friendly physician if you don't already have one.

Honestly, once you get charting and have done it for several months, you'll start to see your own patterns emerge. You'll get comfortable with your own body's rhythms and won't think twice about minor shifts. Your instructor will help you decipher the information and teach you how to determine your peak fertility days. That's the beauty of NFP—getting to know your own body. It's truly empowering!

STOP LISTENING TO EXTREMISTS

The internet is a wealth of information, but it's also a bottomless pit of extremist views. I'm not just talking about naysayers, either. Nor am I just referring to the "trolls," you know—the people who just surf blogs and Facebook looking to start an argument! There are well-meaning people out there who just happen to be... well... a bit over-dramatic! So, when you're on the internet cruising for blogs, web sites, and support groups to help you on your journey, you will inevitably run in to both the "everything is sunny" person, and the "life is horrible" one as well.

"Everything is Sunny" will say that NFP is foolproof and perfect and simple. She will paint a rosy picture of a happy, blissful life wherein you and your partner are always close, intimate, and loving because the simple steps involved in NFP brought you to that place. She may advocate for only one method, or taut the virtues of NFP in general. Be wary—nothing can be that perfect!

"Life is Horrible" will give you a nightmare scenario of marital unrest because of the strenuous, exhausting, and restrictive aspects of NFP. She may talk about fighting and tension and the frustration of abstinence. She'll point to all the reasons it "doesn't work." But of course, we know that for many, many couples, it does work... and well. Don't let her drag you into her dark abyss!

My suggestion is to stop, look, and listen. When you see someone pitching an extreme viewpoint (even and possibly especially if it's glowing), it's time for you to look at it with a critical eye. Listen to what they are saying and ask yourself if they are coming from a place of love, hate, or rationality. Are their intentions good? Are they full of hate, or maybe trying to sell you a product with their smiling happy linguistic skills? Don't be a pushover. Use your judgment when discerning what information you retain, and what you throw away.

The last thing you want is to go into anything with unreasonable expectations. There are going to be challenges that you and your partner will have to face together—periods of abstinence, frustration with interpreting chart data, constant monitoring of your body. You have to go in understanding that it will not always be easy, but that you can find strength in knowing that all of the trials and frustrations will only work toward building a solid foundation for your marriage, and will bring you and your partner closer.

It's easy to be in love when everything in life is going well. Love is cheap on easy street! But it's through the trials of life that you strengthen your bond with your partner and deepen your relationship in ways that "happy times" cannot. So, when things get tough—not just in your NFP process, but in all aspect of life together-- it helps to take a step back and reframe the situation. Don't think of it as a time that just stinks... approach it as a wonderful opportunity to build a better marriage.

FIND A COMMUNITY

Through the ups and downs of this process, it's good to have a community of supportive, knowledgeable people to help you and give you strength, answer questions, and "compare notes." You might find this within your on site or online classes. But if not, don't worry, there are other places to find a community. You might first check with your church (if you have one), because often times support groups are part of their programming.

You can also find many online groups by simply doing an internet search for "NFP Support Groups." Or you could try searching for a group that focuses on your specific method. You can further narrow the search by adding indicators like, "Catholic," "Christian," or "Secular." If you face a particular challenge in your process, you could even further narrow your search by typing that in, such as "Postpartum" or "breast feeding."

Another good resource is Facebook—there are at least a half dozen NFP groups, both open (public) and closed (private), to choose from. For most of these, you must request to join and be approved by a group administrator... but they offer very relaxed forums to discuss a wide range of topics, and can often lead to lasting friendships.

Make sure you read all of the information you can find about any given group prior to joining, so that you know you're finding a good match for you belief systems, methods, and needs.

Last but not least, don't forget your partner! He is there to be your number one support person—that's what makes NFP so special. Lean on him... but not solely on him. He won't have ALL the answers and shouldn't be relied on to be your sole companion.

BE CONSISTENT

NFP only works when you use it accurately and consistently, especially when you're using it to avoid pregnancy. When used precisely, NFP is up to 99%

effective in preventing unwanted pregnancy. New scientific research published in "Science Daily" indicates that multiple-method NFP (such as STM or SHM), used correctly, works equally as well as oral contraceptives when using it to avoid pregnancy.

However, those statistics drop when couples are sloppy in the execution of their chosen method. In fact, the numbers that you read about the usage of NFP as a contraceptive generally reflect all users (including the sloppy ones)—and that number makes NFP seem ineffective with an unplanned pregnancy rate of 24%. But don't be alarmed. As you can see, it's when couples are not being vigilant (as with any birth control method) that unexpected conception occurs.

USE ABSTINENCE TO GET CLOSE

The thing about using NFP as a form of prevention is that there are stretches of abstinence that absolutely must be observed. However, that does not mean that you and your partner can not be intimate during those times. *Let's redefine intimacy not as simply intercourse, but as a deeper understanding of and love for the person you married.*

These periods of abstinence might be a good time to refocus on why you love your partner, on learning and trying what they like to do, understanding their needs and desires outside the bedroom, and bonding over one of the many other aspects of your life together.

Here are a few of the countless ways that you and your partner can be intimate during periods of abstinence:

- Take longs walks together holding hands
- Cuddle up with a movie
- Kiss
- Dance
- Play a sport (team-like softball, or individual-like tennis)
- Take a class
- Cook a meal or bake
- Read a book out loud to each other

- Go out to intimate candlelit dinners

- Play games/cards/video games

- Set aside family time (if you have other children)

- Go on nature hikes

- Complete projects

- Go hot-tubbing or to a sauna

- Get couples massages

- Go to the beach, pool, or on a picnic in the park

- Give each other a massage

- Explore one-another's bodies

- Other non-genital sexual activity

The possibilities go way beyond this list. It's up to you to learn what makes you feel closer to your partner, and what makes them feel closer to you.

KEEP AN OPEN MIND!

While change may be frustrating, it's often inevitable—and it can be exciting! Not only will your reasons for using NFP likely change throughout the course of your relationship, so, too, will your body. You may start out using NFP as a method of birth control... but as your marriage progresses, you could find yourself using those peak fertility periods to conceive!

As you go through life's many changes, your body will react accordingly. You may see your cycle become what looks like "irregular" during periods of high stress, or if you suffer a physical illness. Your cycle will definitely change if you are pregnant, post-pregnancy, and during breast feeding.

By keeping an open mind-- and through the help of your NFP specialist, your doctor, and your community-- you can figure out when it's time to either change methods, adjust your technique, or seek help from a physician. Just remember, by going through the process, you understand your own body so well that you have given yourself a true advantage when it comes time to make a change.

Also, as you become a part of the larger NFP community, each woman will have a different and unique experience. Simply because something is easy or difficult for you, doesn't mean it will be easy or difficult for another... even if she is your same age, height, weight, and so on. Always be respectful of these differences. That way, you can be supportive and also receive the support you need.

TRUST YOURSELF

Knowledge is power, and knowing your own body is truly empowering. Don't be afraid to listen to what it's telling you.

KEEP A JOURNAL

I know you already have a lot to record, but this tip is one that will help you process all the emotions you might be going through, whether you're using NFP to prevent or encourage pregnancy. Any relationship will have its ups and downs, especially new marriages or engagements. You will experience good days and bad days, marital strife and marital bliss. By recording your thoughts and feelings, you not only give yourself a valuable outlet, but you can look back through the pages when you need encouragement.

Sometimes, life gets busy and journaling is the last thing on your mind—but in order for it to be effective, you have to do it. To make journaling an everyday part of your routine, try these simple tips:

Keep your journal handy. You might find yourself sitting on the couch with a few minutes to spare— maybe your toddler fell asleep on your lap or your favorite show is on a commercial break. Whatever the case may be, just five minutes of jotting down your thoughts can be helpful and therapeutic.

Make a gratitude list. Writing down what you're thankful for can be a powerful practice... especially when times are rough. I realize that the last thing you want to do when you're angry and frustrated is to make a list of all the good things in your life, but often that's exactly what you need to pull you out of the darkness. People who make gratitude lists report an increase in happiness... and that's always a good thing!

Get your partner on board. If your partner is also keeping a journal, not only will he experience the same therapeutic effects, but you could use it as a form of communication. By swapping and reading each other's entries (with permission, of course), you can each gain a valuable insight into your partner's emotional state. Effective, respectful communication is the key to a happy marriage!

By incorporating some, or all, of these tips into your routine, you'll find that Natural Family Planning really is a simple practice that incorporates seamlessly into your life. In fact, it will become integral in shaping your relationship and your family... and pretty soon, it will just become second-nature.

SUPPORT FOR USING
NATURAL FAMILY PLANNING

According to the U.S. Center for Disease Control data, only 4.6% of American women have ever used Natural Family Planning—and only .1% currently use NFP as either a form of birth control or as a fertility method to achieve pregnancy.

That's a very small number... but let's look at it as a small elite group of women and their partners who achieve wonderful things by engaging in NFP. While .1% of the female population that falls within childbearing range sounds like a very small number—it's actually close to 5 million women using NFP methods. And of course, that also means about 5 million men. What do they gain—and could you gain—by joining them?

Recently, a large-scale research study was completed on the effects of NFP on marriages and families, in particular. The research was conducted under the supervision of a highly respected statistician, University of Chicago Sociologist with an Economics degree-- Dr. Robert Lerner. Dr. Lerner evaluated the study and compared it with the two largest U.S. government-backed studies of its kind, and he came up with these striking results!

The findings from over 550 detailed surveys of couples using natural family planning methods draw the conclusion that:

Couples using NFP have a dramatically low (0.2%) divorce rate.

While the national divorce rates hovers closer to 50%, this statistic really is quite remarkable!

These couples experience happier marriages.

They are generally happier and more satisfied in their daily life.

They have considerably more marital (sexual) relations.

These couples share a deeper intimacy with their partner than those who use other forms of contraception.

They realize a deeper level of communication with, and understanding of, their partner.

They have relatively large families with many children.

Couples practicing NFP are appreciably more religious and attend church more often.

These families incorporate more prayer into their daily routines.

They rely strongly on the teachings of the Church, the Bible and Almighty God.

They experience greater levels of personal happiness.

These couples tend to have strong traditional, social, and moral views.

The group of people practicing NFP tend to preserve the family unit more responsibly than the other groups.

They are unlikely to have ever had an abortion.

They are unlikely to have ever have lived together outside of marriage.

This is kind of an interesting one-- They are less likely have both partners working full time.

They don't support or engage in sexual relationships outside of marriage.

While more studies are needed to determine whether some of these characteristics are causative or effects of practicing NFP, the results clearly show that people practicing the method have solid family values and happier marriages than the general population. Isn't that a good reason to join the ranks of happy couples all over the country?

ADDITIONAL RESOURCES

Billings Ovulation Method

Mucus only Method

PO Box 2135

St. Cloud, MN 56302

Phone – 651-699-8139

Website: www.boma-usa.org

Other Billings Ovulation Method information

http://www.thebillingsovulationmethod.org/how-does-the-

billings-ovulation-method%E2%84%A2-work.html

Couple to Couple League

Sympto-Thermal Method

PO Box 111184

Cincinnati, OH 45211-1184

Phone - (513) 471-2000

Website:www.ccli.org

Creighton Model Fertility Care System

Mucus only Medical Model

6901 Mercy Road

Omaha, NE 68106

Phone - (402) 390-6600

Website: www.popepaulvi.com

Marquette University Institute for NFP

Sympto-Hormonal Method

P.O. Box 1881

Milwaukee, WI 53201-1881

(414) 288-3854

Website: http://www.marquette.edu/nursing/NFP

REFERENCES

Archdiocese of St. Louis

http://archstl.org/naturalfamilyplanning/page/different-methods

United States Conference of Catholic Bishops

http://www.usccb.org/issues-and-action/marriage-and-family/natural-family-planning/what-is-nfp/index.cfm

Utah Department of Health Maternal and Infant Health Program on NFP

http://health.utah.gov/mihp/natural_family_planning.htm

Familydoctor.org on NFP

http://familydoctor.org/familydoctor/en/prevention-wellness/sex-birth-control/birth-control/natural-family-planning.html

Medicine.net on Natural Methods of Birth Control http://www.medicinenet.com/natural_methods_of_birth_control/page4.htm

The Roman Catholic Diocese of Harrisburg, Pennsylvania
http://www.hbgdiocese.org/family-life/marriage-and-family/natural-family-planning/history-of-the-church-contraception/

Natural Family Planning Fact Sheet
http://www.hhs.gov/opa/pdfs/natural-family-planning-fact-sheet.pdf

Center for Disease Control: Statistics on National Family Planning
http://www.cdc.gov/nchs/nsfg/key_statistics/n.htm#natural

Wilson, Mercedes Arzú. Rate Comparisons Between Couples Using Natural Family Planning & Artificial Birth Control. (4 March 2001) Physicians for Life.

Natural Family Planning Method As Effective As Contraceptive Pill, New Research Finds. ScienceDaily. (21 February 2007) http://www.sciencedaily.com/releases/2007/02/070221065200.htm

ABOUT THE AUTHOR

KATE EVANS SCOTT is the author of the Amazon Bestselling cookbooks The Paleo Kid, Paleo Kid Snacks, The Paleo Kid Lunchbox and Infused: 26 Spa-Inspired Natural Vitamin Waters.

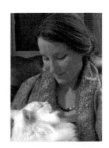

Ever since she turned a new leaf in her twenties, Kate has had a passion for finding alternative health modalities to offer her family and friends while enjoying the ride of self-discovery along the way.

Kate and her husband Mark live in Oregon with their two spirited children.

MORE BY KATE

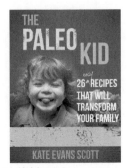

Available Now on Amazon

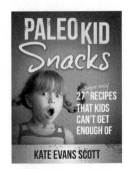

Available Now on Amazon

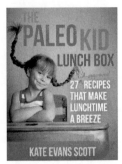

Available Now on Amazon

MORE BY KATE

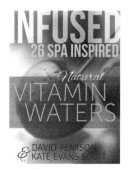

Available Now on Amazon

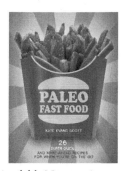

Available Now on Amazon

VISIT:

www.KidsLovePress.com

FOR MORE GREAT TITLES ON

HEALTHY LIVING!!

Printed in Great Britain
by Amazon.co.uk, Ltd.,
Marston Gate.